Introduction

Welcome to your *Lifeline Emergency First Aid, CPR and AED* course. Throughout this course you will learn the necessary lifesaving skills of Cardiopulmonary Resuscitation. CPR is an emergency procedure that keeps blood and oxygen flowing to vital organs when the heart has stopped beating. You will also learn how to recognize an emergency including Heart Attacks, Strokes, and Choking (foreign-body airway obstruction) patients. Approximately 330,000 people die annually from coronary heart disease before reaching an emergency room in North America. In addition to all of this, you will also learn how to deal with people (1) going into shock, (2) bleeding as well as (3) correct bandaging techniques.

Risk Factors

There are several risk factors for the development of Cardiovascular Disease (CVD). CVD includes all diseases of the circulatory system including acute myocardial infarction (heart attack), ischemic heart disease, peripheral vascular disease, arrhythmias, hypertension (high blood pressure), and cerebral vascular disease (stroke). CVD begins when fatty deposits, like cholesterol and cellular debris, accumulate in the inside of the arteries. As the yellowish substance builds, the arteries become narrower and less blood flows through them. As this procedure continues the heart has to work harder to pump the blood through the narrow arteries. The decisions you make every day in our life may increase our chances of developing CVD.

Controllable Risk Factors

1. Drinking Alcohol - Some studies have shown moderate use of alcohol will reduce the risk of heart disease. If you drink, limit your consumption to less than two drinks per day. One drink is considered 1-350ml beer @ 5%, 1-50ml oz of liquor

@ 40%, or 1-150ml glass of wine @ 12%. Do not binge drink.

2. Being Overweight - Being overweight is one of the most common risk factors as our population's obesity rate is at record highs. Males with a waist circumference greater than 40 inches (102cm) and females with a waist circumference greater than 35 inches (88cm) are at highest risk. The increased weight makes your body produce more blood vessels, which increases the amount of blood your body needs. Thus causing your heart to have to work harder.

3. Stress - Everyone in the world has stress. It is how you deal with your stress that is important. The inability to manage stress has been shown to be a factor in the development of heart disease and stroke. Try to contribute a specific amount of time to partake in any activities you find relaxing. Some activities include: Yoga, walking, reading, having a bath, etc.

4. Lack of Exercise - Being physically active is extremely important for people of all ages. The type and duration of physical activity that each person needs to accomplish daily, varies depending on your age, weight, and physical activity level. Every person needs to be involved in an activity which elevates their heart rate for thirty (30) minutes a day at least five (5) days a week. Regular exercise can improve the strength of the heart muscle; maintain a healthy blood pressure, and cholesterol level.

5. Smoking – Cigarette smoke contains numerous gases and chemicals which are detrimental to your health and the health of others. After quitting smoking, your risk of developing CVD and death decreases dramatically. There are several methods available to help you stop smoking. Please consult with your doctor.

6. High Blood Pressure – Blood pressure is the force exerted by the blood against the walls of the vessels. Hypertension, or

high blood pressure, may cause stroke, heart failure, or kidney failure.

> • *Systolic pressure*, which occurs during the heart muscle contraction, averages about 110 and is expressed in millimeters of mercury (mmHg).
> • *Diastolic pressure*, which occurs during relaxation of the heart muscle, averages about 70 mmHg.

The first stages of hypertension begins at 140/90mmHg. Treatment at this point should be based on diet, exercise, and weight loss, if necessary. People with pressure reading above this range, not responding to lifestyle changes, may require use of medication for treatment.

7. High Cholesterol – There are two different types of cholesterol in our body. High-density lipoprotein (HDL), or "good" cholesterol and Low-density lipoprotein (LDL), or "bad" cholesterol. Through our diet you need to increase our "good" cholesterol and decrease our consumption of "bad" cholesterol.

8. Diabetes – Diabetes is a chronic disorder in which the body fails to keep blood sugar at normal levels because of either the lack of the hormone insulin or the body's inability to use it correctly. The number of people to be diagnosed with diabetes in Canada is expected to reach 3 million by 2010. Some of the long term side effects of diabetes include growth failure in children and adolescents, hypertension, kidney failure, blindness, and amputation.

Uncontrollable Risk Factors

1. Family History – Anyone with a family history of heart disease is at a higher risk of developing the disease themselves. Family history includes not only genetics, but also family habits and lifestyle choices. If the parents in the family eat unhealthy, high fat foods, are overweight, and don't exercise, chances are the children will be following their example.

2. Gender – Heart disease is the leading cause of death for both men and women in Canada.

3. Race – Race and ethnic background may play a part in the development for heart disease. In Canada, aboriginals (both Inuit and native North Americans) have a higher risk of heart disease. New Canadians bring with them cultural and lifestyle habits that will influence their risk of developing heart disease. Over time, the risk will become similar to those of Canadians as lifestyle changes.

4. Age – Increased age is a risk factor for heart disease and stroke.

Anatomy & Physiology

Your heart is a hollow organ which pumps blood through the body. The heart is divided into four quadrants. The top two quadrants are the right and left atrium. The bottom two quadrants are the right and left ventricles. The atrium receives blood whereas the ventricles pump the blood. The flow of blood in the body happens in the order that follows:

1. The right atrium is the chamber that receives the blood returning from the body tissues. This blood is low in oxygen. The superior vena cava carries blood from the head, chest,

and arms; the inferior vena cava carries blood from the trunk and legs.

2.   The right ventricle pumps the blood received from the right atrium into the lungs. The blood is carried to the lungs through the pulmonary arteries.

3.   In the lungs the oxygen exchange takes place. The air you breathe in contains about 21% oxygen. Our body only uses about 5% of that 21%. The air you exhale contains about 5% carbon dioxide and 16% oxygen, which is enough to support life. you breathe air in through our mouth and nose. From there the air travels through the airway, into the lungs and into the alveoli. The alveoli are clusters of tiny air sacs in which the gas exchange takes place. *Once a person stops breathing, their heart will stop in 4-6 minutes. Irreversible brain damage is certain after 10 minutes.*

4.   The left atrium receives oxygen rich blood from the lung in the pulmonary veins. The blood is then pumped into the left ventricle.

5.   The left ventricle then pumps the oxygen rich blood to the entire body giving all the organs and tissues the blood and oxygen they require to survive.

Foreign Body Airway Obstruction

In the conscious adult or child patient:

Ask the person "**Are you choking**?"

If they can breathe or talk, no immediate action is required. Stay close and encourage them to keep coughing.

If the person cannot cough or talk you must act quickly. Tell the person that you are going to help them.

Conscious Abdominal Thrusts

1. Stand behind the person.
2. Wrap your arms around the person, placing the flat side (thumb side) of one fist against the stomach, just above the navel. Place the other hand over top of your fist.
3. Quickly thrust inward and upward in a "J" motion. Be sure each thrust is quick and hard to relieve the obstruction.
4. Repeat until the object pops out or the person becomes unconscious. (We will review what to do if the person becomes unconscious later in the course.)
5. When the object comes out you must advise the person to go to a doctor to get checked to verify there has been no further damage caused by the choking or the abdominal thrusts. They must bring the object with them.

Tall / Short People:

Ideally you want to be the same height as the other person. You may need to get them to kneel down on the ground if they are taller then you. If you are taller than your patient, you may need to kneel on the ground to get down to their height. Then follow steps one (1) to five (5) above in the same order.

Obesity or Pregnancy:

With these people there may a few factors that make it not possible to perform an effective abdominal thrust. It may be that your arms are too short to reach around the person, or that with baby, fluid, and tissue there that you are unable to get the diaphragm area to give an effective abdominal thrust. For these people you must use a chest thrust on them. To provide chest thrusts use the following steps:
1. Stand behind the person.
2. Wrap your arms around their chest, coming from under his / her armpits.
3. Place the flat side (thumb side) of one fist against the sternum bone (breast bone). Place other hand over top of your fist.
4. Pull straight back on the sternum bone about 1 ½ - 2 inches (4-5cm).
5. Continue each thrust until the object is expelled or the person becomes unresponsive. (Unresponsive choking will be covered later in the course).
6. When the object comes out you must advise the person to go to a doctor to get checked to verify there has been no further damage caused by the choking or the chest thrusts.

Individuals in Wheelchairs:

Abdominal thrusts are not effective on a person who is sitting down. If you are able to reach around the chair and the person you may be able to perform a chest thrust following the same steps as the obese or pregnant person. If you are unable to reach around the person because of the chair you will have to perform a chest compression by standing in front of him / her. In this case use the following steps:
1. Place the chair against a wall or have someone firmly holding the chair from behind with the brakes on.
2. Stand in front of the patient crouching down so you are about shoulder level.

3. Place the heel of one hand against the length of the sternum bone. Place the other hand in the same position interlocking your fingers.
4. Compress straight back on the sternum bone 1 ½ - 2 inches (4-5cm). It is best to keep your elbows locked and use your body weight to compress.
5. Continue with the chest compressions until the obstruction is expelled or the person becomes unconscious.
6. When the object comes out you must advise the person to go to a doctor to get checked to verify there has been no further damage caused by the choking or the chest thrusts.

* Be sure to keep your mouth closed and head down while completing this procedure. The object may come out towards you and personal injuries should be avoided.

On Yourself / Home Alone

What would you do if you were at home alone and you starting choking? Lots of people have stated they could try several different techniques on themselves. The average person who is choking may be able to try one or two of these things before he / she passes out. This is what you should do:
1. Call 911
2. Go outside to your front lawn / driveway. The sooner someone sees you the sooner you will get help.

If you are unable to get outside try to make it to your front door and unlock it, try to be in a visible spot. If you are unable to be in a visible spot, as a last resort, break a window in your home. (It is a sign of distress and the police will enter your home and find you.)

Driving Alone

Although this scenario is uncommon, it may be worth thinking about as people are known to eat in their vehicles. you have all heard of someone choking while they were driving and using the door or the trunk to get the object out. These two things will not always work. Unfortunately, there are not universal steps to follow so that others on the road will know you are choking. The best thing you can do is safely pull over to the right hand side of the road. Turn your hazard lights on and **get out** of the vehicle. You should stand at the back of your vehicle and try to flag someone down or use the universal sign of choking (place both of your hands around your neck). If you are standing anywhere else your chances of someone seeing you are greatly decreased, especially if you pass out and become unconscious.

* **Remember**: *Once a person stops breathing, their heart will stop in 4-6 minutes. Irreversible brain damage is certain after 10 minutes.*

Infant - Conscious

Infants are treated differently than adults and children when they are conscious and choking. You will notice when an infant is choking, their skin color will change quickly into a reddish and then a blue color. Their cough will become weak; their eyes may appear big and bulging and may start to water. When this happens take the infant, hold a firm grip on their chin, and hole them upside down. Your arm must be resting on a solid surface, such as your leg or an arm to a chair. This is done so gravity will help remove the object.

1. Start by giving the infant five back blows. Use the heel of one hand and hit the infant between the shoulder blades. Once you have completed five back blows, flip the infant on to your other arm, so they are now facing up.
2. Give the infant five chest compressions. Compression on the middle of their sternum bone, about 1/3 to ½ of their chest. Give five chest compressions.

3. Continue the back blows and chest compressions until the obstruction comes out. The infant will start to cry as soon as they are able to breathe and the obstruction is out.

Infant – Unconscious

Follow these steps if you are alone with an infant:

1. Check for Dangers
2. Determine Responsiveness – With infants tickle the bottom of their feet and talk to them.
3. Open Airway – use the sniffing position – have their nose pointing up to the ceiling or sky, but be sure not to hyperextend their head.
4. Check Breathing – if not breathing give two breaths
   If the first breath does not go in and the chest does not rise, reposition the head and attempt another breath.
5. Start Compressions – give 30 compressions (about 1/3 depth of chest)

After each set of compressions, look in the patient mouth for the obstruction. If you see an object remove it and give two slow breaths, if not continue compressions until the object is expelled.
6. **Continue 30 compressions and 2 breaths cycle 5 times**
7. Go call 9-1-1

*Remember infants are smaller than children. You will not breathe as much air into them or compress as hard on them.

The Heart

The heart is a hollow muscle with the purpose of pumping blood throughout your body. It consists of two sides with four chambers in total. The right side of the heart receives blood low in oxygen as the right side receives blood high in oxygen. The upper chamber of each side of the heart (the atrium) is a receiving chamber. The lower one (the ventricle) is a pumping chamber. The *right atrium* receives blood from the body tissues carried in the veins. The superior vena cava carries blood from the head, chest, and arms. The inferior vena cava carries blood from the trunk and legs. The *right ventricle* receives blood from the right atrium. The blood is then pumped through the pulmonary arteries to the lungs. An artery takes blood from the heart to the tissues. The *left atrium* receives blood from the lungs, which is high in oxygen, through the pulmonary veins. The *left ventricle* pumps oxygenated blood throughout the body. Although the right and left sides of the heart are separated from each other, they do work together as one component.

Cardiac Arrest

The term cardiac arrest means a non-beating heart. When a person has gone into cardiac arrest the best things you can do for them is call 911, start CPR, and apply an AED. (We will discuss the AED later in this course.)

Heart Attack

The death of cardiac tissue (heart) occurs with a heart attack. This happens when there is a blockage in at least one of the coronary arteries in the heart. Blood flow is unable to bypass the blockage and any tissue on the other side of the heart may be permanently damaged.

Angina

Angina occurs in people who have partially blocked or narrow arteries in their heart. Angina attacks usually happen when a person is physically active, under stress, or eats a large meal. The area of the heart which has the narrowed arteries is unable to give the heart an adequate amount of oxygen and therefore, causes pain, pressure, or discomfort. This condition may last up to 15 minutes.

Signs   &   Symptoms

Heart Attack
Pain / Pressure
- In the chest, shoulder, neck, jaw, arm, and back.

Shortness of Breath
- Difficulty breathing

Sweating
- Pale, cool, clammy skin

Nausea
- Indigestion

Fear
- Denial
- Anxiety

Angina
Pain / Pressure
- In the chest, shoulder, neck, jaw, arm, and back.

Shortness of Breath
- Difficulty breathing

Sweating
- Pale, cool, clammy skin

Nausea
- Indigestion

Fear
- Denial
- Anxiety

As you can see the signs and symptoms for Heart Attack and Angina are the same. The only way you are going to know the difference is if the person has been to the doctor before and been diagnosed with Angina. If they have been diagnosed with Angina they should have a medication called Nitroglycerin. You can get their medication for them, but they must take it themselves. **You are NOT allowed to administer medication.** This patient may take one dose, wait five minutes, take a second dose, and wait five minutes. If the signs and symptoms are not gone by the second dose or in ten minutes call 911.

* You must ask the patient if they have taken any Viagra or Levitra in the last 24 hrs, Cialis in the last 36 hrs or anything along those lines of medications. If they have, they CANNOT take the nitroglycerin. These medications can be taken by anyone at ANY AGE.

Stroke

The most common cause of a stroke is a blood clot that blocks the flow of blood to an area of the brain. Another cause of a stroke is a ruptured blood vessel in the brain. The severity of the stroke depends on the vessel in the brain which was affected.

Transient Ischemic Attack (TIA)

A TIA is caused by a temporary blockage of a blood vessel in the brain. It is also known as a "mini stroke." A TIA may last for a few minutes or anywhere up to 24hours without any permanent damage done to the brain. TIA's are a major warning signs of a stroke.

The signs and symptoms that the patient will present may vary depending on the area of the brain that is being affected. As you can see the warning signs for a Stroke and a TIA can be the same. Therefore, you will not know which one the person is having and you will need to call 911 immediately.

Signs and Symptoms

Stroke
Speech problems
- Trouble speaking or understanding speech.

Vision Problems
- Double vision or blurred vision.

Dizziness
- Loss of balance, nausea

Headache
- Severe and unusual

Weakness
- Tingling, numbness, or paralysis on one side of the body.

Transient Ischemic Attack
Speech problems
- Trouble speaking or understanding speech.

Vision Problems
- Double vision or blurred vision.

Dizziness
- Loss of balance, nausea

Headache
- Severe and unusual

Weakness
- Tingling, numbness, or paralysis on one side of the body.

The EMS System

The EMS Systems consist of the following emergency response resources......Police, Ambulance, Fire, Hazardous Materials, and Poison Control. If you are in a situation by yourself you may need to leave your patient to go and call EMS. In most cases you will be sending someone to go and call for you. When sending someone else, be sure you identify them by the clothing they are wearing. Tell them **"go call 9-1-1 and come back, do you understand?"** You want to be absolutely positive that this person is going to call 911 for you. When you call EMS you want to give the dispatcher as much information as possible. They will ask you the following questions:

1. What service do you require? Police, ambulance, fire, etc.
2. What is your name?
3. What phone number are you calling from?
4. What is your location / Address?
5. What is your emergency?

6. What is being done for the patient?
7. What is the patient's gender and approximate age?

Barriers

Barriers are personal protective equipment (PPE). Every person should be using barriers in every emergency situation, even if you know the patient. You must take every precaution to protect yourself from blood and bodily fluids of your patient. Barriers include, but are not limited to gloves, face shields, ventilation masks, gowns, and glasses. Make sure your gloves do not have holes in them prior to putting them on and if you have more than one patient you must change gloves between patients. When purchasing a ventilation mask make sure it is equipped with a one-way valve. You don't want to come into contact with anything coming out of your patient. Barriers can help protect you against, but not limited to:

HIV / Aids	Hepatitis	Respiratory
Infections	Herpes/Cold Sores	Blood
Vomits	Urine	Feces
Chemicals		

D.R. 9.1.1. C.A.B.D

This is an easy acronym to use to remember all the steps to follow in an emergency situation.
D – dangers
R – responsiveness
9-1-1
C – circulation
A – airway
B – breathing
D – defibrillation or deadly bleeding

Dangers

The first thing you want to do in any emergency situation is to look for dangers. Dangers include, but are not limited to fire, electrical, traffic, blood, bodily fluids, glass, needles, gases, lack of oxygen, etc. At this time you should recognize or discover the mechanism of injury to our patient. Car accident, fall, or anything to indicate there may be a neck or spinal injury present. Once you know the scene is safe, you need to determine if the patient is responsive or not.

Responsiveness

To determine response you will firmly tap on the collarbone and shout in both ears. You want to ask the patient "Are you ok? Can I help".

9-1-1

As soon as you discover the patient is unresponsive you need to activate EMS. You may need to leave the patient and go call 9-1-1 yourself but preferably, have someone call for you. Once EMS has been activated you need to assess the airway, breathing, and circulation.

Circulation

The heart is a hollow muscle that pumps blood through the blood vessels. The blood delivers oxygen and nutrients to the cells and carries away the waste products of cell metabolism. Slightly bigger then the size of your fist, this organ is located between the lungs, in the center, but slightly left, of the middle of the chest. The average heart pumps 60-100 beats (times) per minute for adults, 80-100 beats per minute for children, and over 100 beats per minute for infants.

CPR means cardiopulmonary resuscitation. You will be compressing on the heart (cardio) and breathing into the patient (pulmonary) for the purpose of resuscitation (re-starting).

After finding a person who is coconscious and who does not appear to be breathing, you will immediately start compressions / CPR.

Airway

Prior to opening the airway, you need to look into the mouth. If you see anything in the mouth, you must remove it. There are three different techniques used to open an airway:

1. Chin – Lift without the head tilt.

   Place one hand on the forehead. Use the hand closest to the feet and place two fingers on the bony part of the jaw. Be sure not to put pressure on the   soft tissue under the jaw. Using your two fingers pull directly up on the jaw.

2. Jaw – Thrust.

   Place one thumb on each cheek bone. Place two fingers on the angle part on the jaw, just below the ear lobes. Using the thumbs to hold the head still, pull directly up on the jaw.

3. Head – Tilt – Chin – Lift.

   Place one hand on the forehead. Using the hand closest to the feet, place two fingers on the bony part of the jaw. Be sure not to put pressure on the soft tissue under the jaw. Using your two fingers pull directly up on the jaw while putting pressure on the forehead to tilt the head back.

When the airway is clear you must check to see if the patient is breathing.

Breathing

Artificial ventilation is the process of giving oxygen to a person through artificial respirations. The air you breathe in contains 21% oxygen. Of that 21% our bodies only use about 5% and exhales approximately 16-17% oxygen. Mouth-to-mask rescue breathing is therefore the quickest, effective way to provide oxygen to a person who is not breathing.

Because the tongue is the most common cause of an airway obstruction in an unconscious person, you must first open and clear the airway. To do this you can use any of the three ways you have already learned about. Once you have an open and clear airway you want to check for breathing. To check for breathing, **while keeping the airway open**, you place your ear close to the patient's mouth

- LOOK for rise and fall of the chest or diaphragm
- LISTEN for any breathing sounds.
- FEEL for any breath on your cheek.

If the patient is breathing adequately you would place them into recovery position (this will be discussed later.) If the patient is not breathing adequately you must perform artificial ventilations.

Defibrillation / Deadly Bleeding

This is the final step of our acronym for you to complete. If you are giving CPR to your patient then you want to get a defibrillator and attach it to the patient as soon as possible. (The defibrillator will be discussed more in detail later.) If your patient is breathing adequately you will look over the body from head to toe. If there is any major bleeding you will need to stop. (Bleeding and bandaging is discussed in our First Aid course.)

Scenario

You are going for a walk along a pathway in the city and you come upon an individual lying on the ground in front of a bench. What do you do?

Follow the steps of our acronym.

1. D – dangers – Look for anything that may be dangerous in the area
2. R – responsiveness – tap the shoulders and shout in the ears for a response
3. 9-1-1 – if the patient is unresponsive call.
4. C – circulation – start compressions on your patient.
5. A – airway – open the patient's airway and look in the mouth
6. B – breathing – look, listen, and feel for patients breathing. If no breathing is present give two artificial respirations and start continue with 30 compressions at a rate of at least 100 compressions per minute.

Artificial Ventilations

To perform artificial ventilations use the following steps:

1. Place a mask over the patient's mouth.
2. Open the airway using same technique used to check for breathing.
3. Take a deep breath.
4. Pinch the patient's nose closed. (With an infant patient there is no need to pinch the nose. You will cover the infant's nose and mouth with your mouth.)
5. Place your mouth over the valve/opening of the mask, making a tight seal on the patient's mouth.
6. Give one full breath. Once you see the chest rise on the patient stop breathing.
7. Wait until the chest completely falls prior to giving a second breath.

If at any point the air does not go in and the chest does not rise, reposition the head and try again. After two attempts initiate CPR and re-inspect the mouth after each set of compressions.

CPR

Place your hand closest to the patient's head on the center of the chest at the nipple line. Place your other hand other top of that hand. Lock your elbows.

Using your body weight push down on the patient's chest at least 2 inches. These "adult" guidelines are for anyone who has reached puberty. Give the patient 30 compressions. You want to push hard and fast.

30 compressions must take no more than 18 seconds to complete. Once you have completed 30 compressions go back to the patient's head and give 2 full breaths. **Two breaths must be completed in no more than 10 seconds.** Continue this compressions and breathing method until an AED or EMS arrives.

Two Rescuer CPR

Two rescuer CPR is easier for the rescuers. All the steps that you have already learned will stay the same. As you approach the area you still want to make sure the scene is safe for you. Introduce yourself to the other rescuer "My name is _____ I know CPR, can I help?" The next question you want to ask is "Has 9-1-1 been called?" If they reply "no", then it will be your job to call 9-1-1. If they have been called ask the other rescuer what they would like you to do. "Would you like me to take over compressions or breathing?" If you are going to be rescue breathing for someone, make sure you are using a barrier device. **CPR should never stop while having this conversation.** One person will complete 30 compressions, and then the other rescuer will give two breaths to the patient. Continue this sequence until one of the rescuers get tired. When the rescuer gets tired tell your partner that you're tired and switch jobs. The individual who was giving the compressions will now give rescue breaths and the individual who was giving the rescue breaths will now be giving compressions.

Child CPR

There are only a few small differences with children and infants compared to adults. A child is anyone over the age of one, but has not yet reached puberty. The biggest difference is if a child is unresponsive and you did not witness the incident, complete five cycles of CPR prior to leaving and calling 9-1-1. If it was a witnessed collapse, call 9-1-1 immediately. For children you should compress to a depth of about 1/3 to ½ the chest using either one or two hands. You will still be completing 30 compressions and two breaths, but you will not breathe as much air into them and don't compress as hard as you would for an adult. Follow these steps if you are alone with a child…..

1. Check for Dangers
2. Determine Responsiveness
3. Start Compressions – give 30 compressions (about 1/3 – ½ depth of chest)
4. Open Airway
5. Check Breathing – if not breathing give two breaths
6. **Continue 30 compressions and 2 breaths for 5 cycles (or 2 minutes)**
7. Go call 9-1-1

*Remember children are smaller than adults. You will not breathe as much air into them or compress as hard on them.

Infant CPR

There are only a few small differences with children and infants compared to adults. An infant is anyone under the age of one. The biggest difference is if an infant is unresponsive and you did not witness the incident, complete five cycles of CPR prior to leaving

22

and calling 9-1-1. If it was a witnessed collapse, call 9-1-1 immediately. For infants you should compress to a depth of about 1/3 – ½ the chest using two fingers of one hand. You will still be completing 30 compressions and two breaths, but you will not breathe as much air into them as you would an adult or child. Also when dealing with infants you want to cover their mouth and nose to give rescue breaths. Their lungs are very small so all you want to do is give a small breath of air, just enough to see the chest rise.

Follow these steps if you are alone with an infant:
1. Check for Dangers
2. Determine Responsiveness – With infants tickle the bottom of their feet and talk to them.
3. Start Compressions – give 30 compressions (about 1/3 depth of chest)
4. Open Airway – use the sniffing position – have their nose pointing up to the ceiling or sky, but be sure not to hyperextend their head.
5. Check Breathing – if not breathing give two breaths
6. **Continue 30 compressions and 2 breaths for 5 cycles (or 2 minutes)**
7. Go call 9-1-1

*Remember infants are smaller than children. You will not breathe as much air into them or compress as hard on them.

Defibrillation

An Automated External Defibrillator (AED) is a portable device which interprets the electrical activity in the heart (heart rhythm). Each AED has two pads which are placed on the patient's chest. You, the operator, will be required to press the shock button if a deliver shock is advised.

There are two heart rhythms which are most common causes of cardiac arrest. One is ventricular fibrillation (VF). When the heart is in VF it shakes like a bowl of jelly, unable to pump blood to the body. The other heart rhythm is ventricular tachycardia (V-Tac.). In V-Tac the electrical impulses in the heart are going anywhere between 200-300+ times per minute. The heart is unable to pump blood to the body at this rate.

Defibrillation shocks the heart and briefly stops all the electrical activity. This allows the pacemaker in the heart, the SA node, to restart its normal electrical activity.

Chances of survival decreases about 7-10% for every minute that passes while waiting for defibrillation. As soon as a defibrillator is available, attach it to the patient and follow the prompts the device tells you.

*Do Not stop CPR while the AED is being attached.

Main components of an AED
- self-testing feature
- data collection tool
- batteries
- on/off button
- shock button
- audible prompts and alarms
- visual prompts and alarms
- adhesive defibrillation pads and cables

AED Accessories
- scissors for removal of all clothing.
- towel to dry the chest if required
- razor for shaving the chest if required
- mask for protective breathing device
- gloves for protection of bodily fluids

Recovery Position

The recovery position is a position in which you will place a patient who is unresponsive **and** breathing adequately. Use the following steps to place a patient into recovery position.

1. Take the patient's arm closest to you and place it straight up, beside their head, lying on the ground.
2. Take the other arm, bring it across their body, and hold their hand in place cupping their neck with your hand closest to their head. DO NOT LET GO OF THE HAND.
3. With your hand closest to their feet pull straight up on their knee furthest away from you, to use it as a lever.
4. Pull that leg at the knee towards you. Be sure to support the head and neck with one hand.
5. The patient will easily roll onto their side.

* You must make sure the patient's face is towards the floor, resting on their arm or hand. This will prevent their tongue from falling backwards and blocking the airway. Also if they vomit, it will drain out of their mouth and not back into the airway.
Remember unconscious/unresponsive people are like "wet noodles", it is not going to be simple or easy to move them. If you let go of their hand or leg it will fall down to the ground, not stay where you put it.

Ongoing Assessment

Ongoing assessment is performed while waiting for EMS. You must reassess the breathing of your patient, recheck wounds to confirm the bleeding has stopped, and reassess injuries. Things can change very quickly with your patient, so you must always be aware of everything that is happening with your patient.

Considerations Special

Breathing

In some circumstances you are unable to breathe into a person's mouth. You may need to breathe into their nose or into a stoma. If breathing into a person's nose, open the airway using the head-tilt-chin-lift technique. Instead of using two fingers on the chin you will need to use your entire hand to lift up on the chin and keep the mouth closed. While giving slow rescue breaths into the patient's nose, be sure to watch for the chest to rise. Some people breathe through a hole in the base of their throat called a stoma. When breathing into a stoma, be sure to have a tight seal around the stoma and watch for the chest to rise. If you hear air escaping out the mouth or nose, will need to pinch the nose shut and close the mouth with one hand while breathing into the stoma.

Head, Neck, Spinal Injuries

In some situations you may have to deal with a patient who may have a head, neck, or spinal injury. As you approach the situation you will determine the mechanism of injury. If you suspect one of these injuries and the patient is not breathing, use the head tilt without the chin lift maneuver or the jaw thrust to open the airway. Only move a patient when absolutely necessary. If you must move a patient do your best to keep the head, neck, and spine in line with the body.

Late Stages of Pregnancy

If having to perform CPR on a pregnant woman, follow all the steps as all other adults. You will also need to place a pillow, blanket, jacket, or something similar under the right side of the patient, just above the bum on the bottom of their back. This will shift the baby in the uterus, to the left side, and help return blood to the heart.

Exposure to Cold

Hypothermia is abnormally low body temperature of 35C (95F) or less. When a person becomes hypothermic the body has a less need for oxygen due to all body systems slowing down. The body pulls blood from the arms and legs to supply it to core (heart, lungs, and brain). Follow the steps of DR.9-1-1 ABCD. You may need to check for breathing for up to 45 seconds. If the patient is breathing start re-warming by removing any wet clothing and placing blankets over them if possible. If the patient is not breathing, start CPR immediately.

Electric Shock

Your own safety is the most important in situations dealing with electricity. Be sure the power source is off prior to approaching the patient. In some situations you may need to wait for professional help. The best chance of revival for a person who has suffered cardiac arrest due to electrical shock is defibrillation. The patient may have also suffered burns and other injuries.

Drowning

It is possible to revive a patient after being submerged in water for extended periods of time. Once the patient is out of the water and on a firm flat surface follow your
DR 9-1-1 ABCD steps. If you suspect a head, neck, or spinal injury, keep the head and neck supported and in line with the spine while moving the patient. When opening the airway use the jaw thrust maneuver, or the chin lift without the head tilt.

After the Rescue Attempt

The human body deals with two different types of death. Clinical death is when a person stops breathing and their heart stops beating. Biological death occurs when the brain activity stops. You cannot determine when biological death occurs in your patient without specialized equipment. In all cases remember CPR is you giving the patient the best chance of survival and preventing brain damage or biological death. In some situations individuals may feel upset or depressed after a rescue attempt. Some people may need to speak with family or friends about the event which took place. Others may need more specialized help, such as counselors. There are several organizations that offer help to those involved in traumatic events. Be sure to get the help you or your family or friends may need.

Shock, Fainting, Unconsciousness

Shock

Shock is a severe life threatening situation which can lead to death if not recognized and treated quickly. Shock is a medical condition in which there is a lack of oxygen to body tissues. Although there are many causes of shock the exact cause of shock is often unknown. The most common types of shock individuals may have to treat are Anaphylactic, Cardiogenic, Hypovolemic, Septic, Neurogenic or Vasogenic.

Anaphylactic shock is a severe allergic reaction to a substance the individual has an extreme sensitivity to.

Cardiogenic Shock, sometimes called pump failure, is often caused when there has been damage to the heart muscle. If the heart is unable to adequately pump blood to the body, organs and tissues will not receive the oxygen they require to survive. This is the leading cause of shock death.

Hypovolemic shock is due to a decrease in the volume of blood which may occur from severe internal or external bleeding, severe dehydration, or burns.

Septic shock is usually due to an overwhelming bacterial infection in the body.

Neurogenic or Vasogenic shock has two main causes. It is due to an increase in blood vessel dilation. This may occur when an individual has suffered a head or spinal injury, or from medications. Although there is the same amount of blood in the body, the increase in blood vessel size makes it impossible for the blood to be adequately circulated to the organs and tissues.

* Do not confuse fainting with shock.

Signs and Symptoms of Shock
Pale, cool, clammy, skin
Rapid weak pulse
Rapid shallow breathing
May range from alert to disoriented
Nausea
Vomiting
Thirst
Anxiety

First Aid Treatment

Activate EMS (911)
Place the patient in a position of comfort. This may be in a sitting, semi-sitting, or lying position. A person who is having difficulty breathing will not want to lie down, so listen to your patient.
DO NOT give your patient anything to eat or drink. This will cause the blood required to deliver oxygen, and nutrients to the organs and tissues to be pulled away from the core (brain, heart, and lungs) to go to the stomach to aid in digestion. This may also lead to your patient vomiting.
Keep your patient warm, calm, and comfortable.
To get a clear understanding of the severity of shock, let's look at what happens to the body through the stages of shock.

- You come across an individual who has received a severe laceration to their leg.
- The patient's heart starts to beat faster to make up for the blood loss which, in turn causes more blood loss.
- The faster the heart beats the more oxygen the body needs which causes an increase in breathing rate.
- To maintain proper blood and oxygen levels to the core (brain, heart, and lungs), the brain sends a message to pull blood away from the arms and legs.
- As the arms and legs are no longer receiving adequate oxygen tissues are starting to die.

- The brain now sends a message to return blood flow to the arms and legs to stop death of the tissues and cell. Now the vital organs are without adequate blood flow, so the heart tries to beat even faster, and more blood is lost.
- As the vital organs are without adequate oxygen the brain and heart start to die.
- The body's attempt to make up for the loss of blood results in death of the patient.

Fainting

Fainting is a temporary lack of oxygen to the brain. It may be an emotional response to a situation. (This is not always the case). When a patient faints you should lay him/her flat on their back and elevate their feet. You may be required to place a blanket over them to keep them warm, but they are usually fine within a few minutes.

Unconsciousness

There are a number of things that can cause a person to become unconscious. The key things to remember are to call 9-1-1, and assess the patient's airway and breathing. Knowing what caused the patient to become unconscious is not as important and activating EMS and getting them the care that is required.

Bleeding & Bandaging

Blood has three major functions in our body:

1. Transporting oxygen, nutrients, and wastes.
2. Maintaining a constant body temperature.
3. Producing antibodies and defending against infection.

Arteries carry oxygen-rich blood away from the heart to body tissues. Capillaries link arteries and veins; they transfer oxygen and nutrients from the blood to the cells. Capillaries also carry waste products from the cells to the veins. The veins carry waste products and oxygen-poor blood to the heart, lungs, and kidneys for removal of waste and to re-oxygenate the blood.

External bleeding is easy to recognize. You see blood coming out of the body at an injury site. Some of these lacerations may be small from a paper cut or they may be large from a knife. No matter what size the laceration may be you will always treat them the same.

To remember what to do for a bleeding injury, remember the acronym RED. It is easy to remember because it is the color of blood.

> R – rest
> E – elevate
> D – direct pressure

There is no other time that exposes you more to potentially infectious bodily fluids as the time you are dealing with a bleeding patient. Whenever coming to a person who has a bleeding injury the first thing you want to do is be sure you have and are using the proper barriers. Gloves are our best protective device you can use for our hands. You may use glasses to protect your eyes from spurting and splashes of blood.

Once you have your protective barriers on, apply firm direct pressure over the wound. Have your patient sit or lie down, then elevate the injury site. If you do not have any bandages readily available, use your gloved hand.
Ideally you want to use sterile gauze over the wound. If you do not have sterile gauze, use clean dressings.
To keep the dressing in place you may need to apply a pressure bandage. A pressure bandage is something you use to keep the dressing in place with pressure such as wrapping a triangular bandage around the injury site over the dressing or using roller gauze. Be sure not to apply the pressure dressing too tightly, as it may cut off circulation, or too loosely, as it will not stop the bleeding. You should be able to wiggle your pinky finger under the bandaging.

You will notice if you bandage is too tight by checking the skin color, temperature, and pulse, or capillary refill on the extremity below the injury site. If your bandage is too tight it will act like a tourniquet. The use of a tourniquet is strongly discouraged as it has been found to cause more problems than benefits. A tourniquet is a tight object (belt, elastic, bandage, etc.) placed around an extremity to cut off blood flow to the injury spot. The problem with this is the rest of the extremity below the injury site is not receiving any blood or oxygen. Without oxygen the cell and tissues in the extremity will die leading to amputation of the extremity from where the tourniquet was applied.

If your bandage is too loose, the bleeding will continue. Place more dressing over top of the existing bandaging and apply more direct pressure.
If direct pressure does not stop the bleeding, then a pressure point may be used. A pressure point is where the vein lies across a bone close to the surface of the skin. One is the brachial artery, which is located on the inside of the arm just above the elbow in between the muscle. A second pressure point you may need to apply pressure to for the leg is called the femoral artery. It is located across the pelvic bone close to the groin.

Amputation Care: Dealing with the extremity would be the same as any other open wound. Apply direct pressure to the end of the extremity, elevate the extremity, and you would probably apply pressure to a pressure point after applying a pressure bandage. For the pact of the extremity that has been amputated you need to place it in a clean bag, wrap with a towel, and place over ice.
DO NOT place the extremity on ice and DO NOT place ice into the bag. This may cause the tissue of the extremity to freeze or absorb the water from the melting ice which will cause the extremity to swell.

Impaled Object: The initial reaction for someone with an impaled object is to pull it out immediately. The only time you may consider removing an impaled object is if it is obstructing the patient's airway and they are unable to breathe. Removal of the object may cause severe damage and be extremely painful. The wound will not bleed much, if at all, due to the object acting like a plug. Get whatever type of padding material you have available and place it around the object. Be sure not to apply any pressure to the object. Then take any type of triangular bandages, roller gauze, tea towels, belts etc; and tie the padding into place. Again be sure not to apply pressure to the object. Never wrap anything around the object. Any movement of the object will be painful and cause more damage to the underlying tissues.

Nose Bleed: Care for a nose bleed is very simple. Pinch or have the patient pinch their nose and lean forward. Never stuff Kleenex, toilet paper, paper towel, or any similar substance up the nose. It may help with clotting, but as you pull out the tissue, the clot will come out with it and the bleeding will start again.

Internal Bleeding

Internal bleeding may be very hard to detect in some patients. You must think about the mechanism of injury to your patient. Pain, swelling, and bruising are the most common signs and symptoms. Always call 9-1-1 if you suspect someone has internal bleeding.

For More Online Courses Go To

www.LifelineEducationalServices.com

www.ingramcontent.com/pod-product-compliance
Lightning Source LLC
Chambersburg PA
CBHW060017300526
45794CB00003B/1209